CHEMOTHERAPY DIET COOKBOOK

Mary Dixon

TABLE OF CONTENT

CHAPTER ONE

Chemotherapy Diet and Benefits

A chemotherapy diet is not a substitute for medical treatment but can complement it by supporting your overall health during cancer treatment. Here are some guidelines on how to follow a chemotherapy diet with potential benefits:

1. Consult with a healthcare professional: Before making any significant dietary changes, consult with your oncologist or a registered dietitian who specializes in oncology. They can provide personalized guidance based on your specific cancer type, treatment plan, and individual needs.

2. Focus on nutrient-rich foods:

- Incorporate a variety of fruits and vegetables into your meals. These provide essential vitamins, minerals, and antioxidants to support your immune system and overall health.
- Choose lean protein sources such as poultry, fish, tofu, and legumes to help maintain muscle mass and support tissue repair.
- Opt for whole grains like brown rice, quinoa, and whole wheat bread for sustained energy.

3. Stay hydrated: Chemotherapy can cause dehydration, so drink plenty of water throughout the day to stay hydrated. Herbal teas and clear broths can also contribute to your fluid intake.

4. Limit processed foods: Minimize your consumption of processed and packaged foods high in sugars, unhealthy fats, and additives. These can contribute to inflammation and negatively affect your overall health.

5. Manage portion sizes: Pay attention to portion control to maintain a healthy weight and avoid overeating, which can lead to fatigue and discomfort.

6. Control nausea and digestive issues: Chemotherapy often causes nausea and digestive problems. To alleviate these symptoms:

- Eat small, frequent meals throughout the day.
- Choose bland, easy-to-digest foods like crackers, plain rice, and toast.
- Ginger and peppermint tea can help soothe nausea.

7. Include sources of healthy fats: Incorporate sources of healthy fats, such as avocados, nuts, seeds, and olive oil, into your diet to support overall health.

8. Be cautious with supplements: Discuss the use of dietary supplements with your healthcare provider. While some supplements may be beneficial, others can interact with chemotherapy drugs or negatively impact your treatment.

9. Stay mindful of food safety: A weakened immune system during chemotherapy makes you more susceptible to foodborne illnesses. Practice good food hygiene by washing your hands, fruits, and vegetables thoroughly, and avoiding raw or undercooked foods.

10. Listen to your body: Your appetite and dietary preferences may change during chemotherapy. Be flexible and prioritize foods that are easy to tolerate and provide the nutrients you need.

11. Seek support: Join a support group or seek guidance from a registered dietitian who specializes in oncology to help you navigate the challenges of a chemotherapy diet and maintain your overall well-being.

Remember that the goal of a chemotherapy diet is to support your health during treatment, manage side effects, and enhance your overall well-being. It's crucial to work closely with your healthcare team to tailor your diet to your specific needs and treatment plan.

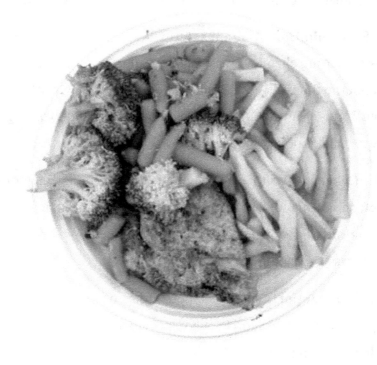

CHAPTER TWO

14-Day Chemotherapy Diet Meal Plan

A chemotherapy diet meal plan should prioritize nutrient-dense foods and aim to manage common side effects like nausea, fatigue, and changes in taste.

Remember that individual dietary needs may vary, so it's essential to consult with a registered dietitian or your healthcare team to create a personalized plan. Here's a sample 14-day chemotherapy diet meal plan to provide you with ideas:

Day 1:

- Breakfast: Scrambled eggs with spinach and whole-grain toast
- Snack: Greek yogurt with honey and berries
- Lunch: Grilled chicken breast with quinoa and steamed broccoli
- Snack: Sliced apple with almond butter
- Dinner: Baked salmon with asparagus and brown rice

Day 2:

- Breakfast: Oatmeal with sliced banana and a sprinkle of chia seeds
- Snack: Carrot and cucumber sticks with hummus
- Lunch: Lentil soup with a side of mixed greens and vinaigrette dressing
- Snack: Cottage cheese with pineapple chunks
- Dinner: Stir-fried tofu with broccoli, bell peppers, and brown rice

Day 3:

- Breakfast: Smoothie with spinach, banana, Greek yogurt, and a dash of honey
- Snack: Trail mix with nuts and dried fruit
- Lunch: Turkey and avocado wrap with a side salad
- Snack: Sliced pear with a handful of walnuts
- Dinner: Grilled shrimp with roasted sweet potatoes and steamed green beans

Day 4:

- Breakfast: Whole-grain cereal with almond milk and sliced strawberries
- Snack: Celery sticks with peanut butter
- Lunch: Quinoa salad with chickpeas, cucumbers, tomatoes, and feta cheese
- Snack: Mixed berries and a small piece of dark chocolate
- Dinner: Baked chicken thighs with roasted carrots and quinoa

Day 5:

- Breakfast: Scrambled tofu with sautéed mushrooms and spinach
- Snack: Edamame with sea salt
- Lunch: Brown rice bowl with black beans, avocado, and salsa
- Snack: Cottage cheese with sliced peaches
- Dinner: Poached cod with a lemon-dill sauce, served with steamed asparagus and wild rice

Day 6:

- Breakfast: Whole-grain waffles with Greek yogurt and fresh berries
- Snack: Sliced cucumber with tzatziki sauce
- Lunch: Spinach and strawberry salad with grilled chicken and balsamic vinaigrette
- Snack: Sliced mango with a sprinkle of Tajin seasoning
- Dinner: Beef stir-fry with broccoli, snap peas, and brown rice

Day 7:

- Breakfast: Smoothie bowl with acai, banana, and granola
- Snack: Cherry tomatoes with mozzarella cheese
- Lunch: Lentil and vegetable stew with a side of whole-grain bread
- Snack: Sliced kiwi with a drizzle of honey
- Dinner: Grilled swordfish with quinoa and sautéed kale

Day 8:

- Breakfast: Overnight oats with almond milk, sliced peaches, and a sprinkle of cinnamon
- Snack: Sliced bell peppers with guacamole
- Lunch: Grilled vegetable and goat cheese wrap with a side of mixed greens
- Snack: Mixed nuts (unsalted)
- Dinner: Baked trout with lemon and herbs, served with quinoa and roasted Brussels sprouts

Day 9:

- Breakfast: Whole-grain English muffin with scrambled eggs, spinach, and a slice of tomato
- Snack: Sliced pineapple with a touch of lime juice
- Lunch: Brown rice bowl with grilled shrimp, avocado, and a cilantro-lime dressing
- Snack: Greek yogurt with honey and a handful of granola
- Dinner: Turkey meatballs with marinara sauce, whole-wheat spaghetti, and a side of steamed broccoli

Day 10:

- Breakfast: Smoothie with kale, banana, almond milk, and a scoop of protein powder
- Snack: Celery sticks with almond butter
- Lunch: Quinoa salad with roasted vegetables and feta cheese
- Snack: Sliced watermelon with a squeeze of lime
- Dinner: Baked chicken breast with a garlic-herb sauce, served with quinoa and sautéed spinach

Day 11:

- Breakfast: Whole-grain pancakes with fresh berries and a dollop of Greek yogurt
- Snack: Cherry tomatoes with mozzarella and basil leaves
- Lunch: Chickpea and vegetable curry with brown rice
- Snack: Sliced oranges with a sprinkle of cinnamon
- Dinner: Grilled portobello mushrooms with balsamic glaze, quinoa, and steamed green beans.

Day 12:

- Breakfast: Scrambled eggs with smoked salmon and whole-grain toast
- Snack: Sliced cucumber with tzatziki sauce
- Lunch: Spinach and strawberry salad with grilled chicken and balsamic vinaigrette
- Snack: Mixed berries and a small piece of dark chocolate
- Dinner: Beef stir-fry with broccoli, snap peas, and brown rice

Day 13:

- Breakfast: Green smoothie with spinach, banana, almond milk, and a scoop of protein powder
- Snack: Edamame with sea salt
- Lunch: Lentil and vegetable stew with a side of whole-grain bread
- Snack: Sliced kiwi with a drizzle of honey
- Dinner: Grilled swordfish with quinoa and sautéed kale

Day 14:

- Breakfast: Greek yogurt parfait with granola, sliced peaches, and a drizzle of honey
- Snack: Sliced bell peppers with hummus
- Lunch: Turkey and avocado wrap with a side salad
- Snack: Sliced mango with a sprinkle of Tajin seasoning
- Dinner: Baked salmon with asparagus and wild rice

Feel free to continue rotating these meals throughout your chemotherapy journey, adjusting portion sizes and ingredients as needed.

Always stay well-hydrated, and remember to consult with your healthcare team or a registered dietitian for personalized advice and any necessary modifications to your diet plan.

CHAPTER THREE

Chemotherapy Diet Breakfast Recipes

1. Nutrient-Packed Breakfast Bowl

Start your day with a nutrient-packed breakfast bowl filled with antioxidants, fiber, and protein to support your body during chemotherapy.

Ingredients:

- 1/2 cup rolled oats
- 1 cup almond milk (or your preferred milk)
- 1 tablespoon chia seeds
- 1/2 cup mixed berries (fresh or frozen)
- 1 tablespoon honey
- 1/4 cup chopped nuts (such as almonds or walnuts)
- Fresh mint leaves for garnish (optional)

Instructions:

1. In a bowl, combine rolled oats and almond milk. Stir in chia seeds and refrigerate overnight or for at least 30 minutes.

2. In the morning, top the oat mixture with mixed berries, drizzle with honey, and sprinkle with chopped nuts.

3. Garnish with fresh mint leaves if desired.

Cooking Time: 5 minutes (plus overnight soaking)

2. Scrambled Tofu with Spinach

This protein-packed breakfast is perfect for a savory start to your day, providing essential nutrients for your chemotherapy journey.

Ingredients:

- 1/2 block of firm tofu, crumbled
- 1 cup fresh spinach leaves
- 1/4 onion, finely chopped
- 1/2 bell pepper, diced
- 1 clove garlic, minced
- 1/2 teaspoon turmeric

- Salt and pepper to taste
- Cooking oil (e.g., olive oil or coconut oil)

Instructions:

1. Heat a little cooking oil in a skillet over medium heat. Add chopped onion and bell pepper, and sauté until softened.

2. Add minced garlic and crumbled tofu to the skillet. Sprinkle with turmeric, salt, and pepper.

3. Cook for 5-7 minutes, stirring occasionally, until tofu is heated through and slightly browned.

4. Add fresh spinach leaves and cook for an additional 2-3 minutes until wilted.

5. Serve hot.

Cooking Time: 15 minutes

3. Banana and Spinach Smoothie

A green smoothie may not sound appetizing, but this one is delicious and packed with vitamins and minerals to boost your energy levels.

Ingredients:

- 1 ripe banana
- 1 cup fresh spinach leaves
- 1/2 cup Greek yogurt
- 1/2 cup almond milk (or your preferred milk)
- 1 tablespoon honey (optional)
- Ice cubes (optional)

Instructions:

1. Place all ingredients in a blender.

2. Blend until smooth and creamy.

3. If desired, add ice cubes for a colder smoothie or honey for added sweetness.

Cooking Time: 5 minutes

4. Avocado Toast with Poached Egg

Creamy avocado and protein-rich eggs make this breakfast a tasty and nutritious choice for your chemotherapy diet.

Ingredients:

- 1 slice whole-grain bread
- 1/2 ripe avocado
- 1 poached egg
- Salt and pepper to taste
- Optional toppings: red pepper flakes, chopped fresh herbs

Instructions:

1. Toast the slice of whole-grain bread.

2. While the bread is toasting, mash the ripe avocado and spread it evenly on the toasted bread.

3. Top with a poached egg and season with salt and pepper.

4. Add optional toppings, if desired.

5. Serve immediately.

Cooking Time: 10 minutes (including poaching the egg)

5. Berry and Greek Yogurt Parfait

A delightful parfait filled with Greek yogurt and antioxidant-rich berries is a quick and nutritious breakfast option.

Ingredients:

- 1/2 cup Greek yogurt
- 1/4 cup granola
- 1/2 cup mixed berries (e.g., strawberries, blueberries, raspberries)
- 1 tablespoon honey (optional)

Instructions:

1. In a glass or bowl, layer half of the Greek yogurt.

2. Add half of the granola and half of the mixed berries.

3. Repeat the layers with the remaining ingredients.

4. Drizzle with honey for added sweetness, if desired.

Cooking Time: 5 minutes

6. Overnight Chia Seed Pudding

Prepare this overnight chia seed pudding in advance for a convenient and nutrient-packed breakfast option.

Ingredients:

- 2 tablespoons chia seeds
- 1 cup almond milk (or your preferred milk)
- 1/2 teaspoon vanilla extract
- 1 tablespoon honey (optional)
- Fresh fruit for topping (e.g., sliced banana, berries)

Instructions:

1. In a jar or bowl, combine chia seeds, almond milk, vanilla extract, and honey (if using). Stir well.

2. Refrigerate overnight or for at least 4 hours, stirring occasionally.

3. In the morning, give it a good stir, top with fresh fruit, and enjoy.

Cooking Time: 5 minutes (plus overnight soaking)

7. Whole-Grain Pancakes with Berries

Whole-grain pancakes loaded with berries provide fiber, vitamins, and a touch of sweetness to your morning.

Ingredients:

- 1/2 cup whole-grain pancake mix
- 1/2 cup almond milk (or your preferred milk)
- 1/2 cup mixed berries (e.g., blueberries, raspberries)
- Cooking spray or oil for the pan
- Maple syrup (optional)

Instructions:

1. In a bowl, mix the pancake mix and almond milk until well combined.

2. Gently fold in the mixed berries.

3. Heat a non-stick skillet or griddle over medium heat and lightly grease with cooking spray or oil.

4. Pour small portions of the pancake batter onto the skillet to make pancakes.

5. Cook until bubbles form on the surface, then flip and cook until golden brown on both sides.

6. Serve with a drizzle of maple syrup if desired.

Cooking Time: 15 minutes

8. Apple Cinnamon Oatmeal

A warm and comforting bowl of apple cinnamon oatmeal is a soothing breakfast option that provides fiber and energy.

Ingredients:

- 1/2 cup rolled oats
- 1 cup almond milk (or your preferred milk)
- 1 small apple, peeled, cored, and diced
- 1/2 teaspoon ground cinnamon
- 1 tablespoon honey (optional)
- Chopped nuts for garnish (e.g., almonds or walnuts)

Instructions:

1. In a saucepan, combine rolled oats, almond milk, diced apple, and ground cinnamon.

2. Cook over medium heat, stirring occasionally, until the oats are soft and the mixture thickens (about 5-7 minutes).

3. If desired, drizzle with honey and sprinkle with chopped nuts before serving.

Cooking Time: 10 minutes

9. Peanut Butter and Banana Sandwich

A simple and satisfying sandwich that combines the creaminess of peanut butter with the natural sweetness of bananas.

Ingredients:

- 2 slices of whole-grain bread
- 2 tablespoons natural peanut
- butter (without added sugars)
- 1 ripe banana, sliced

Instructions:

1. Spread peanut butter evenly on one slice of bread.

2. Layer the banana slices on top.

3. Place the second slice of bread on top to create a sandwich.

4. Cut in half and enjoy.

Cooking Time: 5 minutes

10. Spinach and Mushroom Omelette

This protein-packed omelette filled with spinach and mushrooms is a savory and nutritious breakfast choice.

Ingredients:

- 2 large eggs
- 1 cup fresh spinach leaves
- 1/2 cup sliced mushrooms
- 1/4 onion, finely chopped
- Salt and pepper to taste
- Cooking oil (e.g., olive oil or coconut oil)

Instructions:

1. In a bowl, whisk the eggs until well beaten. Season with salt and pepper.

2. Heat a little cooking oil in a non-stick skillet over medium heat.

3. Add chopped onion and sliced mushrooms and sauté until softened.

4. Add fresh spinach leaves to the skillet and cook until wilted.

5. Pour the beaten eggs over the vegetables and cook until set, lifting the edges to allow uncooked eggs to flow underneath.

6. Fold the omelette in half and slide it onto a plate.

7. Serve hot.

Cooking Time: 10 minutes

These breakfast recipes provide a variety of options for your chemotherapy diet, from sweet to savory, and they are designed to help you maintain your energy levels and overall well-being during treatment.

Chemotherapy Diet Lunch Recipes

1. Quinoa and Chickpea Salad

This quinoa and chickpea salad is packed with protein, fiber, and essential nutrients, making it a perfect lunch option during chemotherapy.

Ingredients:

- 1 cup cooked quinoa
- 1 can chickpeas, drained and rinsed
- 1 cup cherry tomatoes, halved

- 1 cucumber, diced
- 1/4 cup red onion, finely chopped
- Fresh parsley or cilantro for garnish
- Lemon vinaigrette dressing (olive oil, lemon juice, salt, pepper, and a touch of honey)

Instructions:

1. In a large bowl, combine cooked quinoa, chickpeas, cherry tomatoes, cucumber, and red onion.

2. Drizzle with lemon vinaigrette dressing and toss to combine.

3. Garnish with fresh herbs.

4. Serve chilled.

Cooking Time: 20 minutes (including quinoa cooking time)

2. Grilled Chicken and Avocado Wrap

A grilled chicken and avocado wrap is a satisfying lunch option filled with lean protein and healthy fats.

Ingredients:

- 1 boneless, skinless chicken breast
- 1 whole-grain tortilla wrap
- 1/2 ripe avocado, sliced
- Lettuce leaves
- Tomato slices
- Greek yogurt or hummus for dressing

Instructions:

1. Grill the chicken breast until fully cooked and slice it into strips.

2. Lay the tortilla wrap flat and place lettuce leaves on it.

3. Add the grilled chicken, avocado slices, and tomato slices.

4. Drizzle with Greek yogurt or hummus.

5. Roll the wrap and secure it with a toothpick if needed.

6. Serve immediately.

Cooking Time: 15 minutes

3. Lentil and Vegetable Soup

A hearty bowl of lentil and vegetable soup provides essential nutrients and can be prepared in advance for easy lunches.

Ingredients:

- 1 cup dried green or brown lentils, rinsed
- 4 cups vegetable broth
- 1 cup diced carrots
- 1 cup diced celery
- 1 cup diced onions
- 2 cloves garlic, minced
- 1 bay leaf
- Salt and pepper to taste
- Fresh parsley for garnish

Instructions:

1. In a large pot, sauté onions, carrots, celery, and garlic until softened.

2. Add lentils, vegetable broth, bay leaf, salt, and pepper.

3. Bring to a boil, then reduce heat and simmer for about 30 minutes or until lentils are tender.

4. Remove the bay leaf before serving.

5. Garnish with fresh parsley.

6. Serve hot.

Cooking Time: 45 minutes

4. Tuna and White Bean Salad

A tuna and white bean salad is a protein-packed and easy-to-make lunch option for your chemotherapy diet.

Ingredients:

- 1 can white beans, drained and rinsed
- 1 can tuna in water, drained
- Cherry tomatoes, halved
- Red onion, finely chopped
- Fresh basil leaves, torn
- Lemon vinaigrette dressing (olive oil, lemon juice, salt, pepper)

Instructions:

1. In a large bowl, combine white beans, tuna, cherry tomatoes, red onion, and torn basil leaves.

2. Drizzle with lemon vinaigrette dressing and toss to combine.

3. Serve chilled.

Cooking Time: 10 minutes (no cooking required)

5. Roasted Vegetable and Quinoa Bowl

Roasted vegetables paired with quinoa make a filling and nutritious lunch that's perfect for chemotherapy patients.

Ingredients:

- 1 cup cooked quinoa
- Assorted vegetables (e.g., bell peppers, zucchini, cherry tomatoes, red onion), chopped
- Olive oil
- Salt and pepper
- Fresh herbs (e.g., thyme or rosemary)

Instructions:

1. Preheat the oven to 400°F (200°C).

2. Toss the chopped vegetables with olive oil, salt, pepper, and fresh herbs.

3. Spread the vegetables on a baking sheet and roast for about 20-25 minutes or until tender.

4. Serve the roasted vegetables over cooked quinoa.

5. Drizzle with a little olive oil if desired.

6. Serve hot.

Cooking Time: 30 minutes (including quinoa cooking time)

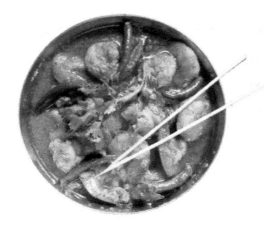

6. Turkey and Avocado Salad

A turkey and avocado salad is a protein-packed and refreshing lunch option that provides essential nutrients during chemotherapy.

Ingredients:

- Sliced turkey breast
- Mixed greens (e.g., spinach, arugula, and romaine lettuce)
- 1/2 ripe avocado, sliced
- Cherry tomatoes, halved
- Cucumber slices
- Balsamic vinaigrette dressing

Instructions:

1. Arrange mixed greens on a plate.

2. Top with sliced turkey, avocado, cherry tomatoes, and cucumber slices.

3. Drizzle with balsamic vinaigrette dressing.

4. Serve cold.

Cooking Time: 10 minutes (no cooking required)

7. Egg Salad Lettuce Wraps

Egg salad lettuce wraps are a light and protein-rich lunch option for those on a chemotherapy diet.

Ingredients:

- Hard-boiled eggs, chopped
- Greek yogurt or mayonnaise
- Dijon mustard
- Chopped celery
- Chopped red onion
- Salt and pepper
- Large lettuce leaves (e.g., iceberg or butter lettuce)

Instructions:

1. In a bowl, mix chopped hard-boiled eggs, Greek yogurt or mayonnaise, Dijon mustard, chopped celery, and red onion.

2. Season with salt and pepper to taste.

3. Spoon the egg salad mixture onto large lettuce leaves.

4. Roll the leaves to create wraps.

5. Serve immediately.

Cooking Time: 20 minutes (including boiling eggs)

8. Quinoa and Black Bean Bowl

A quinoa and black bean bowl is a protein-packed and fiber-rich lunch option that can be customized with your favorite toppings.

Ingredients:

- 1 cup cooked quinoa
- 1 can black beans, drained and rinsed
- Corn kernels (fresh or frozen)
- Sliced avocado
- Salsa or pico de gallo
- Chopped fresh cilantro (optional)
- Lime wedges

Instructions:

1. In a bowl, combine cooked quinoa and black beans.

2. Top with corn kernels, sliced avocado, and salsa or pico de gallo.

3. Garnish with chopped cilantro if desired.

4. Serve with lime wedges for squeezing over the bowl.

Cooking Time: 20 minutes (including quinoa cooking time)

9. Greek Salad with Grilled Chicken

A Greek salad with grilled chicken is a refreshing and protein-rich lunch option that's packed with flavor.

Ingredients:

- Grilled chicken breast
- Mixed greens (e.g., romaine lettuce, cucumbers, cherry tomatoes, red onion, kalamata olives, feta cheese)
- Greek dressing (olive oil, red wine vinegar, lemon juice, garlic, oregano, salt, and pepper)

Instructions:

1. Arrange mixed greens, cucumbers, cherry tomatoes, red onion, olives, and feta cheese on a plate.

2. Top with grilled chicken breast.

3. Drizzle with Greek dressing.

4. Serve cold.

Cooking Time: 15 minutes (including grilling chicken)

10. Baked Sweet Potato with Chickpea Salad

A baked sweet potato topped with chickpea salad is a hearty and fiber-rich lunch option for your chemotherapy diet.

Ingredients:

- Sweet potatoes
- 1 can chickpeas, drained and rinsed
- Chopped red onion
- Chopped bell peppers (red, green, or yellow)
- Chopped fresh parsley
- Lemon-tahini dressing (tahini, lemon juice, garlic, salt, and pepper)

Instructions:

1. Preheat the oven to 400°F (200°C).

2. Bake sweet potatoes until tender (about 45 minutes to 1 hour).

3. In a bowl, combine chickpeas, red onion, bell peppers, and fresh parsley.

4. Drizzle with lemon-tahini dressing and toss to combine.

5. Cut open the baked sweet potatoes and stuff with the chickpea salad.

6. Serve hot.

Cooking Time: 1 hour (including baking sweet potatoes)

These lunch recipes offer a range of flavors and nutrients to support your chemotherapy diet. Adjust ingredients and portion sizes according to your dietary preferences and recommendations from your healthcare team. Enjoy your nourishing and delicious lunches!

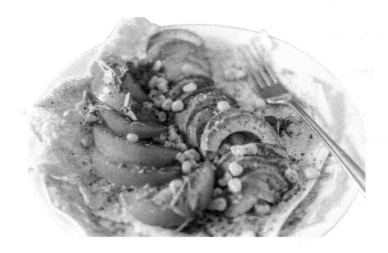

CHAPTER FOUR

Chemotherapy Diet Dinner Recipes

1. Lemon Herb Baked Salmon

Lemon herb baked salmon is a delicious and protein-rich dinner option that provides essential omega-3 fatty acids.

Ingredients:

- Salmon fillets
- Fresh lemon juice
- Fresh herbs (e.g., dill, parsley, or thyme)
- Garlic, minced
- Olive oil
- Salt and pepper

Instructions:

1. Preheat the oven to 375°F (190°C).

2. Place salmon fillets on a baking sheet.

3. Drizzle with fresh lemon juice and olive oil.

4. Sprinkle with minced garlic, fresh herbs, salt, and pepper.

5. Bake for 15-20 minutes or until salmon flakes easily with a fork.

6. Serve hot.

Cooking Time: 20 minutes

2. Grilled Chicken with Quinoa and Steamed Broccoli

Grilled chicken paired with quinoa and steamed broccoli is a well-balanced dinner option that's rich in protein and fiber.

Ingredients:

- Boneless, skinless chicken breasts
- Quinoa
- Broccoli florets
- Olive oil
- Lemon juice
- Salt and pepper

Instructions:

1. Season chicken breasts with olive oil, lemon juice, salt, and pepper.

2. Grill the chicken until fully cooked.

3. Prepare quinoa according to package instructions.

4. Steam broccoli florets until tender.

5. Serve grilled chicken over cooked quinoa with steamed broccoli on the side.

6. Drizzle with additional olive oil or lemon juice if desired.

Cooking Time: 30 minutes

3. Tofu Stir-Fry

Tofu stir-fry is a versatile and plant-based dinner option that's rich in protein and vegetables.

Ingredients:

- Extra-firm tofu, cubed
- Mixed vegetables (e.g., broccoli, bell peppers, snap peas)
- Garlic, minced
- Ginger, minced
- Low-sodium soy sauce
- Sesame oil
- Cornstarch (optional)
- Brown rice or quinoa

Instructions:

1. In a wok or large skillet, heat sesame oil over medium-high heat.

2. Add cubed tofu and stir-fry until lightly browned.

3. Add minced garlic and ginger, followed by mixed vegetables.

4. Stir-fry until vegetables are tender-crisp.

5. In a separate bowl, mix low-sodium soy sauce and cornstarch (if using) to make a sauce.

6. Pour the sauce over the tofu and vegetables and stir until heated through.

7. Serve over cooked brown rice or quinoa.

Cooking Time: 30 minutes

4. Baked Chicken with Roasted Sweet Potatoes

Baked chicken with roasted sweet potatoes is a comforting and balanced dinner option packed with protein and vitamins.

Ingredients:

- Chicken thighs or breasts
- Sweet potatoes, peeled and cubed
- Olive oil
- Paprika
- Garlic powder
- Salt and pepper
- Fresh rosemary (optional)

Instructions:

1. Preheat the oven to 400°F (200°C).

2. Season chicken with olive oil, paprika, garlic powder, salt, and pepper.

3. Place chicken on a baking sheet.

4. Toss sweet potato cubes with olive oil, salt, pepper, and fresh rosemary (if using).

5. Arrange sweet potatoes around the chicken on the baking sheet.

6. Bake for 25-30 minutes or until chicken is cooked through and sweet potatoes are tender.

7. Serve hot.

Cooking Time: 30 minutes

5. Lentil and Vegetable Curry

Lentil and vegetable curry is a flavorful and plant-based dinner option rich in protein and fiber.

Ingredients:

- Red lentils
- Assorted vegetables (e.g., bell peppers, carrots, peas)
- Onion, chopped
- Garlic, minced
- Ginger, minced
- Curry powder
- Coconut milk
- Olive oil

- Salt and pepper
- Fresh cilantro for garnish
- Brown rice

Instructions:

1. In a large pot, sauté chopped onion, minced garlic, and minced ginger in olive oil until fragrant.

2. Add red lentils, curry powder, and chopped vegetables.

3. Pour in coconut milk and enough water to cover the ingredients.

4. Simmer until lentils and vegetables are tender.

5. Season with salt and pepper.

6. Serve over cooked brown rice, garnished with fresh cilantro.

Cooking Time: 45 minutes (including simmering time)

6. Spaghetti Squash with Tomato and Basil Sauce

Spaghetti squash with tomato and basil sauce is a low-carb and vitamin-rich dinner option that's both delicious and nutritious.

Ingredients:

- Spaghetti squash
- Tomatoes, diced
- Fresh basil leaves, chopped
- Garlic, minced
- Olive oil
- Salt and pepper
- Grated Parmesan cheese (optional)

Instructions:

1. Preheat the oven to 375°F (190°C).

2. Cut the spaghetti squash in half lengthwise and scoop out the seeds.

3. Drizzle olive oil, salt, and pepper over the cut sides of the squash.

4. Place the squash halves cut-side down on a baking sheet and bake for 30-40 minutes or until tender.

5. In a saucepan, sauté minced garlic in olive oil until fragrant.

6. Add diced tomatoes and chopped fresh basil. Cook until tomatoes break down and sauce thickens.

7. Use a fork to scrape the cooked squash into "spaghetti" strands.

8. Serve with tomato and basil sauce.

9. Sprinkle with grated Parmesan cheese if desired.

Cooking Time: 45 minutes (including baking the squash)

7. Poached Cod with Lemon-Dill Sauce

Poached cod with lemon-dill sauce is a light and flavorful dinner option that's rich in protein and omega-3 fatty acids.

Ingredients:

- Cod fillets
- Lemon juice
- Fresh dill, chopped
- Garlic, minced

- Olive oil
- Salt and pepper

Instructions:

1. In a large skillet, heat olive oil over medium heat.

2. Add minced garlic and cook until fragrant.

3. Place cod fillets in the skillet.

4. Drizzle with lemon juice and sprinkle with fresh dill, salt, and pepper.

5. Cover and simmer for 8-10 minutes or until the fish flakes easily with a fork.

6. Serve hot with additional lemon-dill sauce.

Cooking Time: 15 minutes

8. Stir-Fried Shrimp with Broccoli

Stir-fried shrimp with broccoli is a quick and protein-packed dinner option that's perfect for busy nights.

Ingredients:

- Shrimp, peeled and deveined
- Broccoli florets
- Garlic, minced
- Ginger, minced
- Low-sodium soy sauce
- Sesame oil
- Cornstarch (optional)
- Brown rice

Instructions:

1. In a wok or large skillet, heat sesame oil over medium-high heat.

2. Add minced garlic and ginger and stir-fry until fragrant.

3. Add shrimp and stir-fry until pink and opaque.

4. Add broccoli florets and continue to stir-fry until tender-crisp.

5. In a separate bowl, mix low-sodium soy sauce and cornstarch (if using) to make a sauce.

6. Pour the sauce over the shrimp and broccoli and stir until heated through.

7. Serve over cooked brown rice.

Cooking Time: 20 minutes

9. Baked Eggplant Parmesan

Baked eggplant Parmesan is a comforting and vegetarian dinner option that's rich in fiber and flavor.

Ingredients:

- Eggplant, sliced into rounds
- Marinara sauce (store-bought or homemade)
- Mozzarella cheese, shredded
- Parmesan cheese, grated
- Fresh basil leaves, chopped
- Olive oil
- Salt and pepper
- Whole-wheat breadcrumbs (optional)

Instructions:

1. Preheat the oven to 375°F (190°C).

2. Brush eggplant slices with olive oil, season with salt and pepper, and bake for 20-25 minutes or until tender.

3. In a baking dish, layer baked eggplant slices, marinara sauce, mozzarella cheese, Parmesan cheese, and chopped fresh basil.

4. Repeat the layers as desired.

5. Top with whole-wheat breadcrumbs for added crunch (optional).

6. Bake for an additional 20 minutes or until bubbly and golden.

7. Serve hot.

Cooking Time: 45 minutes

10. Beef and Vegetable Stir-Fry

Beef and vegetable stir-fry is a protein-rich dinner option that's packed with colorful veggies and flavor.

Ingredients:

- Lean beef strips (e.g., sirloin or flank steak)
- Mixed vegetables (e.g., bell peppers, snap peas, carrots)
- Garlic, minced
- Ginger, minced
- Low-sodium soy sauce
- Sesame oil
- Cornstarch (optional)
- Brown rice

Instructions:

1. In a wok or large skillet, heat sesame oil over medium-high heat.

2. Add minced garlic and ginger and stir-fry until fragrant.

3. Add beef strips and stir-fry until browned.

4. Add mixed vegetables and continue to stir-fry until tender-crisp.

5. In a separate bowl, mix low-sodium soy sauce and cornstarch (if using) to make a sauce.

6. Pour the sauce over the beef and vegetables and stir until heated through.

7. Serve over cooked brown rice.

Cooking Time: 20 minutes

Chemotherapy Diet Snack Recipes

1. Hummus and Veggie Sticks

Hummus and veggie sticks are a nutritious and satisfying snack that's rich in fiber and essential nutrients.

Ingredients:

- Baby carrots
- Cucumber sticks
- Bell pepper strips
- Cherry tomatoes
- Sugar snap peas
- Hummus

Instructions:

1. Wash and cut the vegetables into sticks or strips.

2. Serve with a side of hummus for dipping.

3. Enjoy immediately.

Preparation Time: 10 minutes

2. Greek Yogurt with Berries

Greek yogurt with berries is a protein-packed and antioxidant-rich snack that's both creamy and delicious.

Ingredients:

-   Greek yogurt
-   Mixed berries (e.g., strawberries, blueberries, raspberries)
-   Honey (optional)

Instructions:

1. Spoon Greek yogurt into a bowl or serving cup.

2. Top with mixed berries.

3. Drizzle with honey for added sweetness, if desired.

4. Enjoy chilled.

Preparation Time: 5 minutes

3. Cottage Cheese and Pineapple Cups

Cottage cheese and pineapple cups are a protein-rich and refreshing snack with a sweet twist.

Ingredients:

-   Low-fat cottage cheese
-   Pineapple chunks (fresh or canned in juice)
-   Fresh mint leaves for garnish (optional)

Instructions:

1. In small serving cups, layer low-fat cottage cheese and pineapple chunks.

2. Garnish with fresh mint leaves, if desired.

3. Enjoy chilled.

Preparation Time: 5 minutes

4. Almond Butter and Banana Slices

Almond butter and banana slices make for a creamy and satisfying snack that's rich in healthy fats and potassium.

Ingredients:

- Banana, sliced
- Almond butter

Instructions:

1. Slice a banana into rounds.

2. Spread almond butter on each banana slice.

3. Arrange on a plate and enjoy.

Preparation Time: 5 minutes

5. Trail Mix

Trail mix is a portable and energy-boosting snack that combines a variety of nuts, seeds, and dried fruits.

Ingredients:

- Almonds
- Walnuts
- Pumpkin seeds

- Sunflower seeds
- Dried cranberries
- Dried apricots
- Dark chocolate chips (optional)

Instructions:

1. Mix all the ingredients together in a bowl.

2. Portion into snack-sized bags for easy, on-the-go snacking.

3. Enjoy as needed.

Preparation Time: 5 minutes

6. Sliced Apples with Peanut Butter

Sliced apples with peanut butter are a classic and satisfying snack that provides fiber, vitamins, and healthy fats.

Ingredients:

- Apple, sliced
- Natural peanut butter (without added sugars)

Instructions:

1. Slice an apple into rounds or wedges.

2. Dip each apple slice into peanut butter.

3. Enjoy immediately.

Preparation Time: 5 minutes

7. Rice Cakes with Avocado

Rice cakes with avocado are a crunchy and creamy snack that's rich in healthy fats and fiber.

Ingredients:

- Rice cakes (choose whole-grain for added fiber)
- Ripe avocado, mashed
- Cherry tomatoes, sliced
- Red pepper flakes (optional)
- Lemon juice (optional)

Instructions:

1. Spread mashed avocado onto rice cakes.

2. Top with sliced cherry tomatoes.

3. Sprinkle with red pepper flakes and a squeeze of lemon juice, if desired.

4. Enjoy.

Preparation Time: 5 minutes

8. Frozen Grapes

Frozen grapes are a refreshing and naturally sweet snack that's perfect for cooling down on hot days.

Ingredients:

-   Grapes (red or green)

Instructions:

1. Wash and dry the grapes.

2. Place them in a single layer on a baking sheet and freeze until solid.

3. Serve frozen grapes as a refreshing snack.

Preparation Time: 2 hours (freezing time)

9. Cottage Cheese and Tomato Slices

Cottage cheese and tomato slices are a protein-packed and savory snack that's simple and satisfying.

Ingredients:

-   Low-fat cottage cheese
-   Tomato, sliced
-   Fresh basil leaves (optional)

- Olive oil (optional)
- Balsamic vinegar (optional)

Instructions:

1. Spoon low-fat cottage cheese onto a plate.

2. Top with tomato slices and fresh basil leaves, if desired.

3. Drizzle with a touch of olive oil and balsamic vinegar, if desired.

4. Enjoy.

Preparation Time: 5 minutes

10. Popcorn with Herbs

Popcorn with herbs is a light and savory snack that's low in calories and full of flavor.

Ingredients:

- Popcorn kernels (air-popped or lightly seasoned)
- Fresh herbs (e.g., rosemary, thyme, or basil)
- Olive oil spray (optional)
- Nutritional yeast (optional)

Instructions:

1. Pop the popcorn kernels using your preferred method (air-popped or lightly seasoned).

2. While the popcorn is hot, sprinkle with finely chopped fresh herbs.

3. Optionally, lightly spray with olive oil and sprinkle with nutritional yeast for added flavor.

4. Enjoy while warm.

Preparation Time: Varies depending on popcorn method

These snack recipes offer a range of flavors and nutrients to support your chemotherapy diet. Adjust ingredients according to your dietary preferences and recommendations from your healthcare team. Enjoy your healthy and delicious snacks!

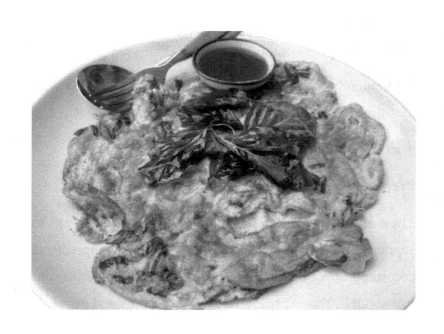

CONCLUSION

In conclusion, a chemotherapy diet is a critical aspect of cancer care that can significantly impact a patient's overall well-being and treatment outcomes. Throughout this exploration of a chemotherapy diet, we have delved into its principles, benefits, meal plans, and recipes designed to provide nourishment, support, and comfort to individuals undergoing cancer treatment.

First and foremost, the primary goal of a chemotherapy diet is to help patients maintain their strength, manage side effects, and support their immune system during the treatment journey.

This is achieved by focusing on a balanced intake of nutrients, including lean proteins, whole grains, fruits, vegetables, and healthy fats, while avoiding or limiting processed foods, excessive sugars, and unhealthy fats. Proper hydration is also emphasized to mitigate the risk of dehydration often associated with chemotherapy.

The benefits of adhering to a chemotherapy diet are manifold. Patients can experience increased energy levels, improved digestion, better weight management, and a stronger immune system. Moreover, a well-planned diet can help alleviate common side effects such as nausea, loss of appetite, taste changes, and mouth sores. By providing the body with the necessary nutrients, patients are better equipped to tolerate their treatments and recover more effectively.

The meal plans and recipes provided serve as practical tools for incorporating a chemotherapy diet into daily life. From nutritious breakfast options to satisfying dinner recipes and convenient snacks, these offerings are designed to cater to different tastes, dietary preferences, and treatment-related challenges. They emphasize fresh, whole foods that can be easily adapted to individual needs.

In essence, a chemotherapy diet is a vital component of holistic cancer care. While it may not replace medical treatments, it complements them by promoting strength, resilience, and overall health. It is essential for patients to work closely with healthcare professionals, including dietitians, to tailor their dietary choices to their specific needs and treatment plans.

Ultimately, a chemotherapy diet is a beacon of hope and support for individuals facing the formidable challenges of cancer treatment.

It empowers them to take an active role in their healing process, offering comfort, nourishment, and a sense of control during a challenging time. By embracing the principles and recipes outlined here, patients can nourish not only their bodies but also their spirits as they navigate their unique cancer journey.

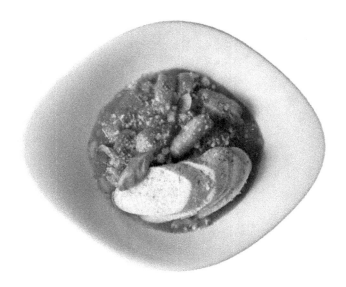

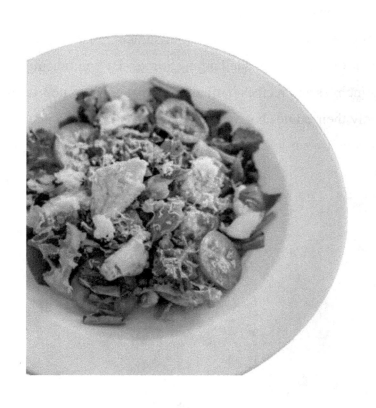